HAZY
SHADE
OF
WINTER

FRANK J. BURROUGHS

FOREWORD BY AMANDA REIMAN, PHD MSW

HAZY SHADE OF WINTER

MY DYSFUNCTIONAL LIFE AS A FUNCTIONAL ALCOHOLIC

Disclaimer: This book is memoir. It reflects the author's present recollections of experiences over time. It is not meant to offer, suggest, or replace medical or professional advice or encourage illegal activity. Although cannabis is "legal" in many states, it remains illegal at the federal level at the time of this publication. This book is simply a means to share with the world what worked for me to end my alcohol addiction and get my life back. I encourage readers to do their own research and make their own decisions regarding their approach to good health, what they put in their bodies, and how they spend their time.

CONTENTS

CHAPTER 1

THE BASEMENT

I came about it honestly. My dad and his dad were both alcoholics, and drunkenness was normal to me. Drinking was my dad's only hobby, and when he wasn't working or sleeping, he was drinking. He used to refer to chores as either a "six-pack job" or a "twelve-pack job." In an effort to conceal his drinking, he would often hide bottles for later or toss his empties in the rafters so no one knew how much he really drank. It's a skill I later perfected. My other grandfather loved his beer too and would always greet me or anyone else on his doorstep with a friendly "Want a beer?" I always accepted and sometimes would empty his fridge.

My mother filed for divorce from my father when I was in third grade, after enduring several years of his drinking and rage. On one occasion, he picked me up and threw me across the room after I sat in his chair when he got up to use the bathroom. On another, he locked my brother and me out of our house and broke our toys as "revenge" for accidentally breaking a lamp. The final straw was when he wrapped his hands around my neck and squeezed after I spilled water in the bathroom while brushing my teeth. I've seen my father do outrageous things while he was drunk, including pissing his pants, picking fights, and screaming at a police officer who was directing traffic while he was driving drunk. Other relatives had problems with alcohol also, which destroyed marriages and good-paying jobs.

Around 1982, the drinking age for beer was still eighteen. I was good friends with several older guys who had graduated from high school the previous summer, so getting beer was never a big problem. I was with these guys the first time I ever got drunk. I was fourteen, and we were all hanging out in my best friend's garage as they worked on his car. I drank five bottles of Miller High Life and absolutely loved the feeling of being fucked up. I also was chewing tobacco at the time, and the nicotine charge took my intoxication to the next level. Just like that, I was hooked. I wanted to get drunk all the time after that.

Pete and I became friends shortly after he moved into our neighborhood during our freshman year in high school. We quickly discovered that we had a mutual appreciation for partying, and it just so happened that his father always had a stockpile of premium beer in his garage. We raided his father's supply of Moosehead and Heineken nearly every weekend until his father said one night to his wife, "Damn, I can't believe I've been drinking that much beer lately." That was just the beginning of what became a notorious life of drunken debauchery.

Despite having the ability to get our hands on beer whenever we wanted it, there was the issue of not having anywhere to drink once we sourced it. After all, we couldn't just sit down in front of our parents and get wasted. We were always tuned in and waiting for someone's parents to go out of town so we could throw a party. While drinking in a warm house or car was preferred, I can remember several very cold winter nights shivering in the back of the neighborhood park while we slammed quarts of beer under cover of trees and darkness.

On the last day of school during my freshman year, I stayed the night at my friend Jim's house to celebrate. Although his mother was going to be home, Jim assured me that she was totally cool with us drinking there. Turns out, not only was she okay with us drinking there, she actually bought us the beer for our last day of school party. I tried marijuana for the first time that night with Jim and his older brother. I remember making out with Jim's younger sister in the dark with Pink Floyd blaring in the room. I got so drunk that night that I tripped and broke my nose on the arm of a couch, giving myself a huge black eye in the process. The next day, I was at a local carryout buying a can of tobacco, and the clerk said to me "It looks like you forgot to duck!"

As my older friends started moving away during my sophomore year, Pete and I became closer. We both shared above-average intelligence, as well as an appreciation for raunchy humor, drinking beer, and pulling pranks. Our idea of fun was getting drunk, soaping cars, toilet-papering houses, or launching snowball attacks on passing school buses. It seemed like every time that we got together, something outrageous would happen, and alcohol would always be involved. It wasn't long before my mother started blaming Pete for all of the crazy shit we'd get into, as if someone was twisting my arm forcing me to drink and get into mischief.

There was one night we went to a professional 9-ball pool tournament together, got drunk and made complete asses out of ourselves. We were laughing, being loud, and heckling the players as they concentrated on their shots. One of the pros, Earl Strickland, bought us a beer in the lobby just to shut us up. I got so drunk that night that I passed out eating a plate of spaghetti when I got home. I woke up the next morning with my mother standing over me with spaghetti all over my white pinstripe dress shirt and the broken plate on the floor.

Our neighborhood was very walkable, and we liberally took shortcuts by hopping fences, jumping ditches, and cutting through backyards to get where we needed to go. None of us had a driver's license yet, and we rode the bus to school. It was a short, twenty-minute trip to and from school, and the bus made several stops in our neighborhood. We would ride in the back and pool our lunch money together to get beer after school, especially on Fridays. It was on the bus where we met Tom, who had something of great value to us: a house to drink in whenever we wanted.

Tom was not a popular person and had no friends. He stood about six feet tall and was overweight and out of shape. He had asthma but smoked cigarettes regularly between puffs on his inhaler. He looked like Lurch from *The Addams Family* with frizzy, unkempt, Brillo pad–like hair. He was the type of guy that I would typically bully and pick on, not spend any time with. But one Friday afternoon, as Pete and I were pooling our beer money together on the bus ride home, the normally silent Tom said to us softly, "You guys wanna come over to my house this weekend? My parents are going out of town." Pete and I looked at each other with wide eyes and didn't hesitate to say, "Hell yes!"

Regardless of whether Tom was a popular guy or not, the fact that he lived within walking distance of us and that his parents were out of town was like hitting the lottery for a hell-raising sixteen-year-old. We knew that we could fill his house with just a few phone calls to our friends for a massive party. And we did just that. We had no idea that his house, especially "The

Basement," would become a notorious hangout and that Tom would soon have more friends than he ever imagined.

Tom lived around the corner from me with his parents and younger sister. I could walk to his house in under five minutes, and Pete could do the same. Tom also had two older brothers who were serving in the U.S. Navy. They lived in a colonial-style home with a full basement. "The Basement" is what became widely known in our school as a safe haven for underage drinking, drugs, and partying. There was a window at ground level that would open just enough to slide cases of beer through the opening, as well as any other contraband that we didn't want to carry through the front door. There was a small bedroom down there that had been Tom's brother Greg's before he joined the Navy. It had a twin mattress on the floor and a mini refrigerator in it…perfect for keeping our beer cold and passing out.

Not only was Tom an asset to us for his house, but he also looked older than his actual age and could purchase beer easily without being questioned, which would be very valuable since my older friends had moved away. There was a small country market located just a few miles from us that we soon discovered was very willing to sell us alcohol without showing proof of age. We started purchasing beer regularly there, often taking turns paying for it so they would all become familiar with our faces.

One night, as we all were partying in The Basement, Tom and I were playing cards when we heard Pete shout out to us from the bedroom, laughing his ass off. Pete had been going through Greg's room and searching through his personal belongings, just for fun. We rushed to the bedroom, and Pete showed us what he had found: Greg's expired passport. Greg was about four years older than Tom, and they looked very similar except the haircut. The passport photo looked spot on. This expired passport was like finding gold for underage drinkers. Even though we rarely got asked for proof of age, now we had something if we needed it. Pete handed Tom the passport, and he took it everywhere. If he was ever carded, he showed it proudly and "became" Greg. As luck would have it, finding that passport was perfect timing.

One Friday after school, the three of us went to the country market to get our weekend beer supply. We had already been buying there for several months without question; however, this time was different. As we entered the store, we saw liquor agents speaking with the owners, who were visibly upset. We carried several cases of beer right past the owners and liquor agents and placed them on the counter. We were asked for identification for the first time, which of course we didn't have…except for Tom. We casually asked what was going on, and the cashier explained that "they got set up and got caught selling alcohol to a minor." Tom stepped up to the cashier and presented his brother's expired passport, which would have made him twenty-two years old. The cashier checked it, and the owners and liquor agents were staring right at us. We purchased several cases of beer, underage, in front of state liquor agents that afternoon, and we were *never* asked for proof of age again at that market. We laughed our asses off all the way back to The Basement.

CHAPTER 2

THE BREW CREW

Sometime during my sophomore year, our school was having a Career Day event where you would shadow someone who worked in a field that you were interested in. I was interested in joining the military and signed up to spend the day at a local recruiting office. A good family friend who I thought very highly of was a retired Marine, and I had no other real interests (other than drinking). The recruiters were handed raw meat when I walked into their office that morning, and by the end of Career Day I had decided to join the Marine Corps.

I was interested in serving in the infantry or military police. I wanted to be a badass—there's no other explanation for wanting those types of jobs. I soon started dressing in military clothing and sporting a "high and tight" haircut. I immersed myself in learning about the military and the Marine Corps in particular. I joined a local Young Marines unit for a brief time, where I learned military history, traditions, and ranks. I memorized General Orders. I was "gung-ho" to graduate early, go to boot camp, and become a real Marine.

I'm not certain how I thought I was going to become a military warrior when I hated authority and spent all of my spare time getting drunk. I knew what the challenge of Marine boot camp would involve, physically and mentally. I guess I figured I'd somehow get my shit together, quit drinking, and get in shape before shipping off to boot camp and miraculously everything would work itself out. In the meantime, I continued feeding my near daily drinking habit.

The regulars who showed up in The Basement started calling ourselves "The Brew Crew" and decorated our school lockers with unique signage. Sometimes we would slam a few beers before school on the side of Tom's house while waiting for the bus, which made for a miserably long day at school. The preferred option, though, was to skip school altogether and hang out at Tom's place while his parents worked. We would each take turns calling the school posing as our fathers: "Good morning. Yes, I'm calling to report my son's absence please. His name is Tom Smith. Yes, uh huh, this is his father, Harold. He's not feeling well today." It worked every time. One day as we were skipping school, drinking beer, and watching *Porky's* on videotape, we heard someone unlock the front door and walk in the house. We nearly shit ourselves as we desperately tried to hide the beer cans. It turned out to be an HVAC repairman Tom's dad had called for service, leaving a key under the mat for him.

It wasn't long before the entire school knew about The Basement and the shenanigans that went on down there. Tom soon started having kids ring his doorbell every weekend, even strangers from other schools occasionally, asking him to buy them beer. Like the idiot he was, he rarely said no and risked his ass for little or no return. Sometimes he'd come back with a free quart or six-pack, sometimes he'd get stiffed. A few years later, Tom was cited for purchasing beer for minors at a local carryout.

One night, Tom's parents were out of town, and I was taking shots out of their liquor cabinet and washing them down with beer. We were on spring break, and I was about to go on vacation with my family the next morning. We had an early flight out and I had not even started packing yet, but I was already well into vacation mode. Pete was over too and was pissed off because someone had stolen his school project for one of his classes and put their name on it. He wanted revenge. Armed with liquid courage, teenage bravado, and a head full of whiskey, we decided to go pay the kid a visit.

We had a sober female friend who lived nearby drive us over to this kid's house. The plan was that Pete would ring the doorbell and confront him about the stolen paper while I hid in the bushes. In the event things escalated, I would pop out and put the fear of God in him. Unexpectedly, after Pete rang the doorbell, the kid's father answered the door. The father must have sensed something was wrong because he wouldn't call his son to the door. Furious, I jumped up from the bushes and confronted the father and threatened him. He locked the screen door, which I then tore off his house and threw in his front yard. He looked terrified and said he was calling the cops. That scared the shit out of us, and we took off back to The Basement.

I got completely shitfaced that night and barely made it home. I fell in a ditch while cutting through yards stumbling home and had water up to my waist. I woke up in the morning feeling like death and looked at my empty suitcase sitting there, and my heart sank. Just then, my mother opened my bedroom door to make sure I was awake and could smell the booze on my breath and permeating my room. She was furious, and I could tell she was very disappointed. She gave me some mints on the way to the airport because I reeked of booze, and it was a very long, miserable day of traveling hungover. On top of that, I barely remembered what happened the previous night, but I knew it wasn't good. I spent most of my vacation worrying about having legal problems when I returned home. Fortunately, I was able to get in touch with Pete later that week on a pay phone, and he said that he was questioned at school about the incident but didn't give up my name. I was extremely relieved and was able to enjoy the remainder of my vacation. I was also looking forward to getting back home to party with my loyal drinking buddies.

My only recollection of high school is drinking. Partying with my buddies was my only priority. Despite my ability to do much better in school, I did just enough to get passing grades with the least amount of effort to graduate. I wasn't interested in getting on the Honor Roll or any classes that involved homework. I'd fill my schedule with study halls, typing, gym, and shop classes. I figured that I wouldn't need physics or calculus in the military because they would teach me everything I would need to know. I basically despised school and would do anything to get out of going, including giving blood. Our school held blood drive events once or twice a year, and my friends and I would always sign up. Why? Because you get out of class for at least an hour, but more importantly, we thought we could get drunk faster after school if we were a pint low on blood. I honestly don't know if that strategy worked, but we always raced to get beer after school on those days to give it a try.

Some of my friends just refused to go to The Basement because either Tom was too creepy or they were afraid of what might happen down there. Regardless, my goal was always to get fucked up and have fun, no matter who I was hanging out with. I had a friend named Rob who was a year older than me and who vomited every time we got together. I remember we were sitting in his car behind a store one night in the middle of winter listening to the new Van Halen *1984* tape and slamming a twelve-pack. I crashed at his place that night, and he was puking his guts out the next morning. On another occasion the next summer, Rob and I drank several beers each before going to see a Def Leppard concert. He puked all over the parking lot while standing in line to enter the arena as I was trying to score us more beer. Another good friend, Billy, was over at my house after school one day because I thought my mother was going to be working late. We each had a twelve-pack and were jamming to the *Animal House* soundtrack when I heard the garage door open and my mother come home early. She walked in, saw what was going on, and proceeded to blister my ass. Billy grabbed his remaining beers and split. He mentioned that incident when signing my high school yearbook.

I had a friend named Ken who lived behind me. His parents were extremely strict, and he was disliked by his stepfather. The parents did strange things like take pictures of the inside of their refrigerator and were constantly pissed off. The kids were given orders not to eat or drink anything after school, and if anything was disturbed, there would be hell to pay. His mother could be heard in the summer when the windows were open screaming at those kids, but especially at Ken. Ken would call me when his parents would be out of town, and I would bring beer over. We would jam to Led Zeppelin and get hammered—usually just the two of us. His younger sister was cute, and sometimes she was there too. I remember kissing her a few times when I was there drinking. I felt sorry for Ken, having to live with such assholes for parents, and he seemed to enjoy the escape from his dysfunctional family life when we got together.

In June 1985, Tom's father offered me, Pete and Tom $500 to paint the exterior of their house. We jumped at the opportunity to earn some cash, and Tom's dad picked up all the supplies. The next weekend, we gathered in Tom's garage, and his father opened up a gallon of paint to show us how to stir it. As he squatted down and started stirring the paint, his nut sack fell out of his shorts and was dangling like a pendulum, only he didn't notice. Pete and I started laughing hysterically. Unaware that his family jewels were on display, he became irritated at our laughter and told us to pay attention. That was a hilarious start to a weeklong project that he most certainly regretted hiring us for.

The job started out well, and the weather was absolutely beautiful. We were excited to be out of school and making good money working outside at the start of our last summer vacation. I had convinced a friend who worked as a bar back at a Holiday Inn to steal a bottle of Jack Daniel's for us. I was in rare form later that week when I downed a twelve-pack of Old Milwaukee and took several slugs of Jack Daniel's. I was on the roof with Pete when I said, "Fuck this!" and launched a gallon of paint off the roof. I climbed down the ladder and threw it on the ground, which stranded Pete on the roof. Pete then launched his can of paint at me as I hopped on Tom's dad's brand-new riding lawn mower and started it up. I was driving in circles around their house and running over the ladder while Pete was screaming at me from the roof. Tom was pleading with me to get off his father's new mower, and I drove over the ladder again. Just then, Tom's father pulled into the driveway. There was brown paint everywhere, including on his brand-new lawn mower. We even painted their bedroom window glass completely brown. Pete and I hauled ass and let Tom face the wrath of his father alone. That was the first of many times to follow that I screwed over an employer.

As I started my senior year, the Marine Corps recruiters were riding me hard to sign the enlistment papers. I was still planning to enlist and perhaps even graduate early to go to boot camp but had not made any written commitment. My mom and dad took me to lunch one day with the goal of convincing me to graduate with my class in June instead of January to go in the Marines. They were worried about me and were not thrilled with the military being my career choice. They hoped that the extra time in school with my friends would change my mind. They made their case pretty convincingly, and since I was starting to have second thoughts about enlisting, I decided not to graduate early. This made my senior year a breeze because I had nearly all the credits I needed to graduate and my schedule was filled with easy classes.

As graduation neared and the recruiters continued to hound me, I decided that I wasn't going to enlist. Needless to say, they were pissed after spending a few years grooming an eager young prospect like me; however, I am certain to this day that I made the right decision not to join the military, as I've never liked being told what to do. I felt relieved after making that decision and soon started working in a local butcher shop after school and on weekends. I became friends with the owners and even dated their daughter for a while. We went to my senior prom together and double-dated with Billy and his girlfriend. I was having the time of my life.

Just before graduation, there was a huge senior party at a nearby quarry. It was a sunny day of swimming, drinking, music, and dancing, and we were all excited for upcoming graduation. The party carried over to someone's house later on, and before we knew it, it was the middle of the night and we hadn't eaten anything. We piled into a friend's car to go steal more beer from Pete's dad and to get some food at Big Boy around 4:00 a.m. On the way back to the party, I wanted to drive my friend's car and asked him for the keys. He reluctantly handed them over and hopped in the passenger seat with the food. Pete was riding in the back and had written "FUCK YOU" in reverse on the condensation of the back window. As I exited the parking lot, I forgot to turn on the headlights, and my friends immediately began yelling at me to turn them on. I was fumbling around trying to find the switch when they then said frantically that there was a cop behind us and to TURN THE LIGHTS ON NOW!

In a momentary lapse of reason, I decided to try outrunning the cops in my friend's piece of shit Comet. Before long, there were two cops behind me with their lights on trying to get me to pull over. I took a hard right turn into the neighborhood where the party was and pulled up on someone's lawn. I had a big dip of tobacco in my lip and spit a huge puddle of tobacco juice on the curb as I stumbled to exit the car. I was totally hammered and had no business being behind the wheel—none of us did. As I stood there wearing my bathing suit at 4:30 a.m., sporting my military haircut, and swaying like a drunken oak tree, I lied to the cops and told them that I was getting ready to ship off to Marine boot camp. I said I couldn't afford to have anything on my record and asked them to let me go. They did. They told my friend who owned the car to drive us back to the party and stay there. That was the first of many close calls while drinking and driving, and eventually my luck ran out.

Just prior to graduation, Tom's parents were out of town, and we were having a huge house party. It had started small, but people started arriving in large waves, which was not unusual. Kids from other schools whom we didn't even know would walk in the house carrying beer and booze. I would never allow this type of party in my own house, but this was not my house and Tom was always a team player. Pete had been over earlier in the evening but had to leave early because he was going on vacation with his family the next day. There were people throughout The Basement, as well as most rooms of the house. People were smoking on the front porch and driveway, and I was beginning to get concerned about someone calling the cops on us about the noise. As I walked up the stairs leading to the bedrooms, which was supposed to be off-limits, I immediately smelled a strong odor of shit and heard the sound of running water. I opened the bathroom door, and there was shit all over the walls and floor. Someone was in the shower, and there was a pair of shitty underwear on the floor. It turns out a classmate of ours, Jorge, shit his pants after drinking too much. I was unfortunate enough to witness the creamy mess smeared between his legs as he drunkenly tried to get cleaned up. Not believing what I just saw, I instantly wished that Pete was still there to witness this hilarious event that became famous at our high school.

I ran down the stairs to find Tom and tell him what happened. Tom was standing in the kitchen with a dozen other people, and I shouted out that "Jorge shit his pants upstairs!" while laughing hysterically. Tom ran upstairs, and others followed into the steamy, fecal fog. Jorge was toweling off but had not succeeded in washing the dung from his inner thighs. He was clearly drunk and very embarrassed, to say the least. Tom got very angry and started ranting that he couldn't believe someone would do that in his house. He went to his brother's room in The Basement and emerged wearing a genuine military-issue gas mask. At this point, I was laughing so hard that tears were streaming down my face. People were running upstairs to see what all the fuss was about and then running back down seconds later, laughing hysterically and pinching their noses. Tom asked me to help get people out of the house; the party was now over.

Jorge disappeared with the crowd making the big exit, leaving us to deal with the aftermath. Tom continued patrolling the house with his gas mask donned, still fuming about the mess that Jorge created for him. As I continued drinking beer in the kitchen with a few other guys, Tom came back downstairs and was now wearing rubber gloves in addition to the gas mask, pinching what appeared to be Jorge's shitty underwear. We immediately decided that we would drive over to Jorge's house and stuff them in his mailbox for his parents to find. We did just that, and I had the honor of sticking them in the box and putting the flag up. As you might guess, this story quickly spread throughout the school, and Jorge was the butt of all poop jokes, no pun intended. Somebody pinned an adult diaper on the wall in the school cafeteria with the caption, "For Jorge's next party!" I'm sure he wanted to switch schools after that, but we were too close to graduation. Jorge left for college a few months later, where I am certain he never told that story to anyone.

In the few short years that we hung out with Tom, we would throw hundreds of parties scaling from small poker games to a house full of more than a hundred drunken teenagers. I graduated with my class in June, as my parents wished, so I could participate in all the "fun" things that most kids do their senior year instead of running off and joining the military. I went to home football games, dances, and even my Senior Prom, and

I got drunk before every one of them. I even drank five beers before my senior picture was taken, and I think about it every time I see the photo: a seventeen-year-old version of me sporting a suit, a crew cut, and an alcohol-induced glow. Drinking gave me the social lubrication I was looking for and was now my favorite pastime. By the time I graduated, I could easily drink more than a case of beer in a night.

CHAPTER 3

PLAYING THE GAME

Shortly after graduation, my good friend Billy and another guy from school were killed while driving drunk. I saw both of them just hours before the collision and had been invited to tag along for the night. I could smell the alcohol on their breath when I ran into them at an electronics store. My Guardian Angel was looking out for me when I turned down their offer because they didn't have a prayer. They had been both been drinking and ran a stop sign that was partially blocked by tree limbs. They were T-boned by a tractor trailer, ejected, and killed instantly. I served as a pallbearer at Billy's funeral, and we got drunk in honor of our dead friends later that night. It was a sad, shocking loss, but unfortunately it didn't serve as a deterrent to my reckless lifestyle.

Just prior to Billy's death, I was dumped by my girlfriend, who was the daughter of my boss. I was devastated. I had become very close to her and had been welcomed into their family. I drank beer and played pool with her father and was often invited over for dinner. They felt like an extension of my own family. I initially was going to quit my job to get away from the situation, but her father convinced me to stay. He told me to "always keep business and personal life separate." I decided to continue working for him and expressed an interest in learning how to cut meat. He said he was willing to train me, and I started coming in on my own time to learn the meat cutting trade. Four months later, he sold the store. The new owner

21

kept me on payroll but started screwing with my hours, so I quit.

I had a few short stints working at a hotel and grocery store before taking a job at a warehouse. It was physically demanding work and miserable when hungover, which was most of the time. I met a new group of friends that liked to party, and we would sometimes meet for pizza and beer before work. There was drive-thru carryout around the corner from the warehouse, and we would hit it occasionally and have a few cold ones on our lunch break. It was the perfect job for a nineteen-year-old who didn't care about anything except getting shitfaced.

One time, we rented a limousine and took it to Canada to the strip clubs because the drinking age was still only nineteen. We were in Michigan heading to the border, and we all had to take a piss, so we told the driver to pull off at an exit. Instead, he just pulled to the shoulder, and we all came piling out to take a squirt on the side of the major highway. Just as we were all relieving ourselves, someone yelled, "Cops!" As soon as I turned my head, blue lights were flashing and a female voice yelled, "Put that goddamn thing back in your pants!" It was a Michigan state trooper who had been following behind us and was now interrogating the driver. The trooper told us to "go back to Ohio" but let us go. We continued to Canada anyway and were ejected from the strip club later that night when one of my drunken friends blew on the genitals of a dancer. We all got tossed out. On the way home, we were all passed out except one guy who continued to drink heavily. We stopped at the border checkpoint and were asked by the customs agent, "Are you bringing anything back to the United States from Canada?" My friend who was still drinking laughed and said, "Oh, nothing but a bunch of hard-ons!"

I started dating a young lady from work and spending less time with my drinking buddies. She lived with her parents, and every time I showed up, I had a twelve-pack with me. She didn't drink very much, and we didn't have much in common. We argued a lot, especially when I was drunk, and she quickly got tired of all the rock star partying. Her parents got sick of me passing out in their basement and leaving bottles everywhere and eventually banned me from staying over. I woke up the morning of my twenty-first birthday in the cab of my truck, parked in front of their house after getting smashed the night before. Many of my days began in front of their house, with the morning sun beaming through my windshield cutting through the stale, boozy air. I'm sure they were thrilled. We eventually got married and were separated a year later after I launched a full basket of clothes at her in a drunken rage, knocking the thermostat off the wall. Thankfully, we had no children, and it was a relatively clean, two-page divorce.

After about a year of working at the warehouse, I grew tired of the physical labor and working in extreme temperatures. I started exploring becoming, of all things, a police officer. My grandfather was a retired cop, and it was a paramilitary field, which I thought I would like. I enrolled in the Criminal Justice degree program at a local community college and was sponsored by a small-town police department to attend the academy. I would work at the warehouse during the day and go to the academy at night. Then I'd usually go to my girlfriend's house and drink beer or have a few at my favorite bar.

Despite my drinking habit, I graduated near the top of my academy class and soon became a sworn police officer. I became just as gung-ho about police work as I had been about the military when I was in high school. I wanted to be on a big-city police department SWAT team or on a paddy wagon crew busting heads. At the same time, I always found it extremely hypocritical and ironic that I enjoyed trolling the streets looking for intoxicated drivers to arrest. I drove drunk all the time when I was off duty and was quickly becoming known as a lush to those I worked with.

I had been working on two small departments trying to make ends meet. After about a year of this, it was becoming apparent that landing a full-time position at a large agency like I wanted would be more difficult than I had planned. As luck would have it, a luxury hotel that Pete had been working at offered me a full-time security position, which I accepted. I liked the convenience of not having to work two jobs to make a living, and I was able to wear a suit to work every day. I got to meet interesting people from all over the world, including rock stars and celebrities. I was working downtown where all the action was and really enjoyed the job. I was promoted to night manager within a few months and had become a protégé of my general manager, who wanted to see me succeed.

Unfortunately, I still had that pesky little alcohol habit that gnawed at all of my ambitions. While I would play the part of a sharp-dressed hospitality executive on the clock, it would be an entirely different story when the whistle blew. There was another hotel next door that had a rooftop bar on the nineteenth floor. This was a very popular late-night spot for hospitality workers and locals, and it offered a spectacular view of the downtown skyline and waterfront. It was not unusual for me to get off work at 11:00 p.m. and go get ripped on the nineteenth floor until closing time at 2:30 a.m. If I was going to be working an early shift the next day, I would often stay in a "blackout" room in my hotel, which is a room taken out of service for a minor maintenance issue. But instead of going to bed when I got off work, I would go to the nineteenth floor for "a couple beers" and party with my co-workers until the wee hours of the morning. I'd drink, watch the clock, and announce, "This is my last beer" several times before finally stumbling back to my room much later than intended. I am certain that there were times that my hangover was very apparent to my general manager and others after staying the night on the property.

The beautiful thing about my position was that I always had a master key, which gave me access to the entire hotel, including all guest rooms. I would print a room report at the start of my shift that lists all occupied rooms, as well as blackout rooms. After a full patrol of the property, I would often unlock one or more rooms on the blackout list and enter. It was not unusual to find a security agent or maintenance guy already in the room kicking back, watching TV, or taking a nap. Blackout rooms were a secret perk of the job known only to maintenance, the bell staff, and security and were fantastic places to take a load off or nurse a hangover.

Other perks of having a master key included the ability to make great tip money. There were always guests who didn't want the party to end and were more than willing to pay for more alcohol. My key opened everything, including liquor storage rooms. Occasionally, horny couples seeking romance would ask me to unlock the Jacuzzi Spa after hours for a "private visit" and would tip very well for me to simply turn the key and open the door for an hour. I'd even use my master key to enter the Presidential Suite on the night shift just to take a dump. I figured since my position presented me a choice between the filthy employee restroom in the basement of the hotel or the Presidential Suite, I might as well take a shit in style.

I had worked at this hotel for about a year when I was recruited by a competitor hotel for the same position. I was offered a considerable pay increase, and I jumped at the opportunity. I gave a two-week notice to my boss, who initially took the news well. Rather than fulfilling my agreed-upon notice, however, I started leaving work early and screwing off even more while I was there. My general manager found out and called me at home to tell me I was no longer needed and to please return my keys. I took a week off before starting my new job at the other hotel. A few months later, I was fired for insubordination after being told that I was needed on the Fourth of July but never showed up. I knew that I'd likely get fired for it but didn't really care. I wanted to party downtown and watch the fireworks with my friends. I was fired on the spot the next day.

At twenty-four, I landed a high-paying union job on an auto assembly line and began drinking before and during work. I started going to my favorite bar before my afternoon shift for a liquid lunch and kept a cooler of beer on ice in my truck for breaks and commuting. We were allotted fifteen minutes for meal breaks, and rather than eat, I would fire down four cans of beer in the parking lot and smoke a cigarette to mask the smell. After work, I'd pick up a forty-ouncer for the drive home and drink until I passed out in my recliner. Or I'd go to the bar and drink until last call and then drive home with one eye shut.

One Friday night at work, some co-workers asked me to join them at a nearby bar when we got off to celebrate a friend's birthday. It didn't take much arm twisting to persuade me to join them for "a couple beers." By closing time, less than four hours after getting off work, I had drank at least six shots of Jack Daniel's and chased it down with at least as many draft beers. I said goodnight to my friends and jumped in my car to head home. I was only a few miles from my apartment, and despite the amount I had drank, I felt fine to drive the short distance. It had started raining lightly, and there was virtually no traffic at that early hour. As I slowed and signaled for a turn, headlights bore down in my rearview mirror, and then the night sky lit up with blue. As I'd feared, the fast-approaching car was a state trooper.

It didn't take long for the officer to smell the booze, perform a mobile breath test, and place me under arrest for driving under the influence. The trooper stopped me for driving sixty-two in a fifty-five-mile-per-hour zone, a minor offense usually overlooked during daylight hours. But in the wee hours of the night, law enforcement will use even small offenses to initiate traffic stops, which often results in a drunk driving and/or drug arrest.

I was handcuffed and taken to the nearest police station, which happened to be in my hometown. As I was led in, another officer met us to perform the official breathalyzer test. I recognized him from the police academy a few years earlier—we had been in the same class together. He recognized me, too, calling me by name as he prepared to perform the test. I couldn't have been more embarrassed. The trooper's suspicions were quickly confirmed when my breath sample registered almost twice the legal limit. My license was seized immediately.

At the end of the day, my decision to drink and drive that night cost me thousands of dollars, three days of my life spent incarcerated, and, worst of all, the loss of driving privileges for more than six months. My car insurance provider, which I'd been with for ten years, dropped me instantly, forcing me to switch to an expensive high-risk policy. I was only allowed to drive straight to and from work, with no stops in between. I had to get rides to go grocery shopping and stopped going to the gym. As much an inconvenience as my arrest was, though, I knew full well that I was long overdue for a DUI. I had been drinking and driving regularly since high school. My luck had simply run out, but as my mother correctly reminded me, I was still in a much better place than my dead friend Billy.

It wasn't long before I found myself in what was referred to as "The Program" at work, an escalating disciplinary procedure for excessive absences or tardiness. I often called off work, either to drink or because I was too hungover, and this kept me in various stages of The Program at all times. After a "rolling" ninety-day period, if no further infractions incurred, you were allotted more unexcused "grace" days before going to the next step in The Program. When one had mastered The Program to the point that he knew exactly when a grace day became available, that was called "Playing the Game."

One night, I was trying to get a pass from my foreman to leave early and go drinking. He had already let a few guys go, and I was nagging him to let me go as well. It was Friday night, and the bar was calling my name. He finally turned to me and said, "What, you want a favor? Don't come to me looking for any fuckin' favors, buddy!" I was very surprised at his reaction and asked him what his problem was. He looked me in the eyes and said, "You want to know what my problem is? It's because you play the game, and you're pretty fucking good at it."

CHAPTER 4

THE DRUNKEN BOSS

Imet my second wife in a crowded bar one Friday night when she and a friend sent a round of drinks to my table. She was pretty, adventurous, had a business degree, and was quickly climbing the corporate ladder. I was a hard-drinking, cigarette-smoking factory worker with no career path, had been arrested the previous month in a DUI, and was getting rides for six months while my driver's license was under suspension. Somehow this didn't scare her away. We hit it off and started dating immediately. I moved into her apartment the next month after my apartment manager gave me a final warning about my loud music and parties. We got engaged, bought a house together, and were married the next summer.

The monotony and repetition of factory work was mind-numbingly boring and constantly left me thinking about an exit strategy. I was tired of working for other people and wanted to be my own boss; however, I had no idea what I wanted to do or how to get there. Early one Sunday morning, we received a phone call from my in-laws, who told us about a lucrative opportunity to take over an established family business. It was a small grocery store in New England that had been in my wife's family for decades. It was a real money maker, and the current owner was retiring. Always up for adventure and ready to roll the dice, we decided to become entrepreneurs. We flew up to tour the business and met with the owners. We ended up making an offer, which was accepted. Within two months, we had quit our good-paying jobs, sold our house, cashed out our retirement accounts, and moved across the country to start a new life and take over the business. The risk paid off very well. After a terribly rough start, including a crippling ice storm and numerous equipment breakdowns, cash was rolling in faster than I could spend it, and it wasn't long before I became very comfortable in my newfound success. I had the ability to come and go as I pleased, to drink whenever and wherever I wanted, and I had the income to do it. We built a home, bought new cars, and vacationed at posh resorts in the Caribbean and Mexico. A few years later, my wife became pregnant with our first child. We had the outward appearance of a fun, successful young couple.

Despite my perceived success, my drinking continued to worsen. I began hiding bottles in my glove box or garage to drink later for a quick "pick-me-up." I would pass out in restaurants at the table, sometimes before we had even been served, to the horrid embarrassment of anyone with me. If I drove to the "big city" about an hour away for errands, I'd always pick up a six-pack and a few mini bottles for the drive home. I didn't care if my employees or customers smelled the booze on my breath and rarely tried to mask it. I began showing up later for work every day, if at all. Who was going to say anything? I was the boss—or at least one of the bosses.

My wife, the other boss, decided that she'd had enough of my bullshit, and on a bright sunny morning just after our daughter's second birthday, she told me that she wanted a divorce. I was shell-shocked. Despite my drinking habit, we had never fought or argued and had the outward appearance of a happy, successful couple. My family and friends were in disbelief. I got completely shitfaced that night and stayed in a motel. I woke up the next morning incredibly hungover, with an overwhelming sense of impending doom and desperation. I was hoping that it had all been a terrible nightmare, but I knew it was real. There were warning signs I had missed or ignored, and now it was happening. I wanted a drink that morning more than anything in the world, but I knew that would only make matters worse. I decided to quit drinking on the spot to try to save my marriage, keep my family together, and be a better business partner.

My marriage didn't make it, but I managed to stay sober for five months, the longest period I had gone without alcohol since I was a kid. This was just long enough to get through a particularly nasty divorce—one that, if I had continued to drink while going through, would have cost me everything. Instead, I stayed away from the bottle, kept my wits about me, and eventually negotiated a six-figure buyout for my half of our business. I obtained joint custody of our daughter and a generous visitation schedule. I was feeling great physically, had lost weight, and was dating a woman I liked in southern Maine.

I had started talking to a counselor once a week to help with the stress and anxiety of the divorce, as well as the alcohol dependency. She strongly suggested that I attend Alcoholics Anonymous meetings regularly, as most counselors do. I reluctantly went to a few meetings but never felt comfortable there. We lived in a small town where everyone knows everyone, and they definitely knew me. I recognized some of the faces in the meetings—a few were even customers of mine—and remember thinking that the entire town would know I was in AA. I don't know why I cared, as the whole town already knew I was a drunk.

One evening, just before the divorce was finalized, I decided to go to an old hangout for chicken wings, but in the back of my mind, even before walking in the door, I knew I was going off the wagon. Things were going so well for me that I figured I could handle a few cold ones to celebrate. As I was seated in the booth, my mind was racing. "Don't do it! Don't do it!" I placed an order for a dozen hot wings and a bottle of beer. The waitress soon returned with an irresistibly frosty bottle neatly wrapped in a cocktail napkin. I took a good haul of the ice-cold beer. It tasted strong and bitter after not drinking for five months, but the more I drank, the better it tasted. In a matter of about an hour, I destroyed five months of hard-earned sobriety with six bottles of beer and drove home with a glow on.

On the day of my divorce, I flew to Cabo by myself to celebrate. I got totally destroyed the night before my flight and barely made it to the airport. I started drinking Bloody Marys in the airline club in Atlanta and was shitfaced by the time I arrived in Mexico. A fellow passenger whom I met on the plane and her husband helped me through immigration, and we shared a taxi to our resorts. I continued to drink throughout the day and nearly was arrested after making an unwanted advance on a female hotel employee. Later that night in the hotel bar, I flirted with a married woman sitting with her husband, who wasn't very appreciative of my drunken forwardness. I slept for nearly twenty-four hours, and I hadn't eaten. I felt like death, and I clearly wasn't handling the divorce well. I decided to fly home the next day before I ended up getting my ass kicked or in a Mexican jail. I checked out of the hotel and took a taxi to the airport. I started drinking again on the flight home and slowly started feeling normal again.

CHAPTER 5

ARMED AND DANGEROUS

With the divorce behind me and in search of a new life, I moved to Charleston, South Carolina, to be near the ocean, palm trees, and the warm, salty breeze. I bought a new house and a new convertible. I bought a new hot tub as a divorce present to myself and had hopes of filling it with several cute southern belles. I had plenty of money in the bank and had no one to report to. I began drinking full time again and had no idea what I was going to do for future work or income—a recipe for disaster. I became a regular at a few local beach bars, where my favorite drinks were poured the moment my car entered the parking lot and were refilled with a nod. I began living the life of a rich, drunken beach bum.

I met a woman with three kids who was going through a divorce. I wasn't physically attracted to her, but I didn't know anyone else in town and she was more than interested in me. She didn't drink at all and didn't seem to mind that I did, so she conveniently became my designated driver and showed me the town. One morning, in what must have been an inebriated fit of insanity, I asked her if she wanted to move in with me. She immediately accepted, and soon there were five heads living under my roof. That lasted only a year, after I caught her oldest daughter stealing cash from my bedroom. I told them to move out, and she ended up renting a townhouse around the corner, which was convenient for me, since we then became "friends with benefits."

I had the travel itch and started taking frequent trips to the Caribbean and to visit family. I attained "status" annually with my preferred airline and was often upgraded to first class, where the free-flowing drinks eliminated the need to smuggle miniature bottles in my carry-on. A membership to the airline's VIP lounge ensured complimentary booze between connections and personal reservation assistance, as well as a quiet, upscale alternative to noisy terminal bars. I began amassing stamps in my passport from exotic locales such as the British Virgin Islands, Anguilla, and the Grenadines and have been shitfaced in some of the most stunningly beautiful destinations in the Caribbean. I'd max out my duty-free liquor limit, which would always include sneaking a bottle or two of Havana Club Cuban rum in the mix, instead of cigars. On one trip, I purchased a $5,000 duty-free Rolex in Grand Cayman, mailed the documents to myself in a Halloween card and wore it back to the States without declaring it to customs. I was drinking and spending like a drunken sailor, but I was spending my own money and buying my own drinks.

Despite my best intentions to start another business or find a job that I enjoyed, having lots of cash in the bank and no one to report to made it way too easy to ignore. After more than a year had gone by since getting divorced and losing my sole source of income, I decided to return to law enforcement work with hopes of getting some stability back in my life. I thought that maybe the camaraderie of other police officers, preferably not alcoholics, might help steer my life back on track. I applied to several departments and received an offer after a lengthy application process. I attended the police academy in Columbia,

South Carolina, for nine weeks, and despite continued boozing while in the academy, I managed to graduate near the top of my class.

The South Carolina Criminal Justice Academy operates Monday through Friday, and recruits return home on the weekends. The first four weeks of the academy were the worst. During that time, we were not allowed to leave the premises, even after classes were finished for the day. They are the most challenging to pass due to the legal coursework, driving, and firearms qualifications. Police departments across the state lose more potential officers during those first four weeks than any other. A score of 70 percent is required to pass, and if a recruit fails a test a second time, he or she is sent home. It is then up to the employing department to decide whether or not they will allow them to return, or "recycle." It is for this reason that recruits were strongly encouraged to study hard the first month and were not allowed to leave the academy after class. If you could get through the first month, you were then granted permission to leave in the evening to go out to eat, run errands, and so on. Or to go find a new watering hole.

My hopes of getting sober and quitting drinking again to give my police career a chance never materialized. After receiving my initial job offer, I continued to drink daily all the way until I started the academy and didn't start exercising at all. I completed the first four weeks without difficulty and would drink like a Viking on my weekends off. Once we were allowed to leave the academy in the evening, I would drive my marked police car to a nearby restaurant and drink several beers and shots before eating dinner. I was fortunate enough to be able to afford this luxury, as most of my fellow classmates on a police recruit salary would eat dinner prepared by prisoners at the academy or pick up fast food. I'd return to the barracks hammered a few hours later driving the same marked police car, hoping like hell that I didn't get pulled over on my way back.

All of my fellow classmates knew that I got drunk every night; they could smell the booze on my breath. One time I received a small cut on my hand during defensive tactics training. The cut wouldn't stop bleeding, and my training partner blurted out something smartass about my blood being too thin from drinking too much. The instructor pulled me aside to look at the wound. She asked me if I was anemic because the small cut continued to bleed. I am not. My ability to heal wounds had become greatly diminished, and the difficulty getting the bleeding to stop was an indicator of liver problems resulting from decades of heavy drinking. I knew it and she likely knew it, but not much else was said. Those who knew me well enough to know how much I drank didn't need to ask.

I wasn't the only one with addiction problems training to be a South Carolina police officer. I had become good friends with a fellow classmate who worked for a department near my home. He had the distinctive drawl of growing up in the Upstate and was funny as hell. He also popped Percocet like candy and struggled with anxiety over the vigorous, continuous academy tests. I had no trouble with the academics and helped him pass the coursework. Just prior to the firearms qualification, he was really stressing out and was afraid he was going to fail the test. He asked me to shoot a round or two into his target to increase his chances of qualifying. I declined, but not because I didn't want to help him or that I was afraid of being caught. I simply wanted to try to shoot a perfect score, and that would be impossible if I dropped a few rounds into his target. He barely passed, and I shot a nearly perfect score.

While I maintained my alcohol habit discreetly, or tried to, there were other recruits in my class who liked to party and raise hell. They were typically younger guys in their early twenties, and most of them worked for the Anderson County Sheriff's Department. They would get drunk at nearby strip clubs until just before curfew and return to the barracks blitzed. As we neared graduation, a rumor circulated that a few of the Anderson County guys had screwed some strippers in the back of their marked police cars. It is my understanding that recruits at the South Carolina Criminal Justice Academy are no longer allowed to leave at all during the entire program. I wonder why?

I lost ten pounds during my stint in Columbia and was recognized at graduation for high academic achievement. My second attempt at a career in law enforcement didn't last very long though. I bounced around a few different departments before deciding that I really had no interest in being a police officer. I hated being told what to do, and my alcohol habit made my dangerous job more dangerous. I found the job to be very negative and depressing because most interactions with the public are an enforcement action or a response to a crisis. In an angry moment after getting a write-up from my supervisor for missing work on New Year's Day, I quit my department without notice. I knew that I'd never get another police job again, but I didn't care. I wanted to work for myself again and not be on someone else's terms.

CHAPTER 6

FLYING HIGH TO ROCK BOTTOM

After a few dating disasters, I met my current wife—my life partner and soul mate—on the internet. Our first date was at a bar. She liked to drink, travel, and hang out at the beach, and soon she became my drinking buddy and travel companion at thirty-eight thousand feet. Our first trip together was to Barbados, where we drank Banks beer and Mount Gay Extra Old with locals at the Oistins Fish Fry and roadside rum shops. Next was a road trip to Key West, a boozy adventure that will never be forgotten. Somewhere on the ceiling of a Duval Street bar is a one-dollar bill inscribed with our names and the proud declaration, "We don't drink anymore. We don't drink any less either!" Our travels led us to some of the most private islands and experiences in the Caribbean. Combined with rum, sunshine, and a sea as clear as Bombay Sapphire, it was the tropical playground seen in Corona commercials. We got married the following year on the beach at the Sullivan's Island Lighthouse and honeymooned in Grand Cayman.

Despite all the fun in the sun, a financial storm was brewing on the horizon. Outstanding investment returns were initially offsetting the cash I was blazing through, but those great returns ended when the recession started in 2008 and the stock market lost half its value. We had just sat down at the Acme

Cantina on the Isle of Palms and ordered a round when we looked up at the TV and saw that the Dow Jones had plunged more than 700 points. I wasn't aware yet of the exact impact this would have on my investments, but I was certain it wasn't good. It was also a great reminder that I really needed to get my shit together and that spending money in bars wasn't the best idea. We had one more round of drinks anyway, paid our tab, and headed for the house. It was time for some financial belt tightening.

While my net worth plummeted, decades of alcohol abuse were starting to manifest. I had always been a very functional drunk, able to push through hangovers and get my work done, but it was becoming increasingly difficult. The more than two thousand calories I was consuming daily in alcoholic drinks had pushed my weight to more than three hundred pounds. The excess weight contributed to high blood pressure, as well as severe back and knee problems. I had no energy, and my sleep was restless and disturbed. I'd never sleep more than a few hours at a time after initially passing out and often woke up drenched in sweat. I kept Gatorade on my nightstand to combat the "hot pipes"—extreme dehydration from a long day's booze consumption—and made frequent trips to the bathroom, further disrupting my sleep. Nausea, vomiting, and dry heaves were becoming a daily ritual, and I once developed pancreatitis after a week of hard partying in Aruba. I consulted my doctor when I returned, and blood work was ordered. It turned out that my pancreatic enzymes were off the charts, and I was warned to quit drinking immediately and permanently or risk dying from pancreatitis. This was an attention-getter, but it didn't stop me.

For years, I had slowly been losing sensation in my toes and feet, but it had gotten considerably worse. I usually walked around barefoot or in flip-flops, and the lack of foot protection and sensation in my feet often led to small cuts that developed into ulcers that wouldn't heal. I consulted a podiatrist about an open and persistent sore the size of a pencil eraser on my big toe. He examined my feet, checked my reflexes, and performed a sensory test. He was noticeably concerned with my severe lack of sensation. He asked if I was diabetic—I am not. After that, it wasn't long before he asked if I drank alcohol and how much. I don't remember exactly what I told him, but I never really tried to hide the fact that I was a big drinker. This was the first time I heard the word *neuropathy*. He said that the numbness and lack of feeling in my feet was likely caused by alcoholism, and he warned that continued drinking would worsen the neuropathy, my ability to heal wounds, and my health in general. I dismissed his advice and was irritated that he didn't have a quick fix for the sore on my toe.

My attempts to return to some semblance of a career were always short-lived and sabotaged by my drinking and poor work ethic. Inevitably, I would become bored, or the demands of an employer would interfere with my drinking schedule and I would move on to greener pastures. Admittedly, I've always hated being told what to do and have a horrible track record working for others. Landing jobs was never difficult, but keeping them and not quitting was always a challenge.

Eventually, a regional supermarket chain offered me an entry-level management position at a salary that exceeded anything I'd been able to earn since owning my own business. This came along at the perfect time, and I was excited to once again try to get my life together. Two months into the new position,

I was sent out of town on the company dime for a week of mandatory training. I checked into the hotel on a Sunday afternoon with a cooler of beer and bottle of Jägermeister and quickly found the nearest bar and package store for future reference.

On Wednesday evening that week, a group of us from the training class met at a Mexican restaurant for drinks and dinner. I had already been priming up in my room with several beers and shots and switched to top-shelf margaritas and tequila at the restaurant. I eventually ordered food but didn't eat, got extremely fucked up, and stumbled back to my room to pass out. When the alarm went off at six o'clock the next morning, my head was splitting, and I felt like death warmed over. I hit snooze several times until finally deciding that it wasn't worth the misery to get out of bed and face the day. Later in the morning, a co-worker I had been out with the night before called, checking why I hadn't shown up, although he knew why. He said I should show up after the break for lunch. Determined not to let another opportunity go down the drain, I dragged myself out of bed, got a shower, and showed up for the afternoon class. I apologized to the instructor for missing the morning session due to "oversleeping" and assured him it wouldn't happen again. Another co-worker who had been drinking with us didn't show up at all, so the rumor mill was starting to churn. Rather than risk word getting back to my boss, I decided to call him and tell him what happened. He wasn't happy, but he didn't fire me either.

I completed the training, returned to my store, and was later promoted to a department management position. I put in long, labor-intensive days on my feet and rewarded myself at quitting time with a chilled twenty-two-ounce can of beer in the parking lot before making the short drive home, where a plethora of booze awaited. I was only able to maintain this pace of "work hard, drink hard" for a brief time before I was back to "playing the game" with extended medical leaves for exaggerated or fabricated problems and requests for time off.

I bruised my ribs after falling down drunk at a friend's Christmas party and used the opportunity to take the holidays off by getting a doctor's note for the injury. My boss was livid. He knew my game, knew it was bullshit, and put me on notice for excessive absences. I walked out of his office with my tail between my legs, wished him a sarcastic Merry Christmas, and booked a flight to visit family for the holidays.

I was scheduled to return to work on January 2, so I chose to fly home on New Year's Eve. Always well prepared, I started drinking in the U.S. Airways Club in Philadelphia before my flight home. I had packed five or six mini bottles of 92-proof Sailor Jerry Rum in my carry-on bag in anticipation of a long travel day. I always made certain that I had a plan in place to be as "self-sufficient" as possible regarding my alcohol supply. In the event of a delay, cancelation, or schedule change, I wanted to have some booze on hand and not be at the mercy of an expensive airport bar or limited stock on a plane. I recall the TSA agent snickering about them when my bag was screened that morning. I later downed them and a few complimentary draft beers in the club while waiting for my connection. I boarded my last leg and had a few more beers in-flight. I was shitfaced by the time I landed and took a cab home. My wife and I drank all night and into the next day. I don't remember much of New Year's Day other than having Chinese food delivered at some point.

When I got to work the next morning, I looked and felt like creeping death. I had dealt with hangovers since I was in high school, but this was way beyond any I'd ever experienced. I was exhausted and dehydrated, and my anxiety was through the roof. My puffy, red face was streaming sweat, and my hands were trembling. I felt like a ragdoll, and my heart was pounding out of my chest. I knew there was no way I'd get through the day without collapsing. I hid from my boss—one look at me and he'd instantly know I was totally fucked up. I'm certain I reeked like stale booze, as it oozed from my pores, sweat, and breath. I had been on the most intense bender of my life and was about to crash.

In a decision that I soon came to regret, I walked out on my good-paying job that morning. I snuck out, really, so as to not be seen or confronted. I knew I would be fired for it, but at the moment, I saw no other way. This was the best opportunity I'd had since my divorce, and my decision to abandon it so I could go home, get a drink and collapse in bed became my personal "rock bottom."

I still had some money in the bank, so there wasn't an immediate financial emergency, but I knew this was *bad*. I would have to tell my wife that I walked out on my job, and she'd know the reason. Hell, she'd even been drinking with me, but she could turn it off. I could never turn it off until the booze ran out (which I never allowed to happen) or until I passed out (that happened every night).

The next few weeks are a blur, as I continued the worst bender of my life. My boss called me once or twice, conversations I only vaguely remember, but I believe he offered me a chance to save my job if I'd go in and talk to him. My pickled brain dictated otherwise. Rather than embrace his offer for help, perhaps even receive company-paid alcohol abuse treatment, I decided to celebrate my newfound "freedom" with a road trip to Key West. It wasn't the "Duval Crawl" I was hoping for though. My stomach was so raw and irritated from heavy boozing and a bad diet that I couldn't hold anything down, and my anxiety was unbearable—the only relief was more booze and Ativan. I would have to force through my first few drinks of the day before I'd start to feel right again. I returned home from the Florida Keys sick, depressed, unemployed, and out of options.

CHAPTER 7

"HE'S DYING"

O n January 29, my anxiety was sky high, and I felt as if my life had unraveled. My good job was gone, my drinking was out of control, my health was failing, and I was as depressed as ever. I remember thinking that even if I'd won the lottery, it would not have made me a happy man. I realized that no amount of money, houses, cars, or vacations would improve my life or bring me true happiness because I was addicted to alcohol. My life had become completely unmanageable, and I had evolved into a chronic alcoholic. I knew that if I didn't make a change, I would die from my alcohol addiction.

I sat in my recliner for hours that morning, telling myself, silently, that I had to quit drinking. I debated whether to quit right then or to aim for a target day. As much as I understood the urgency of quitting, the thought of the withdrawal and anxiety that was going to follow was enough to at least consider delaying the inevitable.

Oddly enough, the thought process alone—of realizing and admitting the extent of my alcoholism—started lifting my spirits. Simply admitting that my drinking was totally out of control and that I needed help somehow gave me a sense of calm and relief. Later that day, I told my wife, with tears streaming down my face, that I had decided to quit drinking and was going to get help to make it happen.

I decided to check myself into the hospital to safely detox. Quitting cold turkey can be dangerous and I wasn't taking any chances. I was given Valium to help with withdrawal and anxiety, and I didn't have any problems other than mild trembling in my hands. I was admitted for seventy-two hours and walked out feeling 100 percent better than when I went in. After three decades of alcoholism, denial, and failed sobriety attempts, I decided to enter an intensive outpatient chemical dependency program.

Blood work was ordered to check for liver damage, and daily piss tests were part of the program. One of the tests run, called GGT, is used to detect liver or bile duct disease and monitor for alcohol abuse. The normal range for this test is 0–51 units per liter of blood. My reading was 881, the highest reading the head counselor had ever seen. He asked for permission to share this with the people in our group. I consented, and when he shared my results the next day, I distinctly remember him saying the words, "He's dying."

Thankfully, that reading returned to normal after a few months of sobriety. I consider it a miracle that I didn't destroy my liver after the abuse I'd put it through for so many years. I finished the treatment program without missing a day. That program taught me a good deal about myself and alcoholism, including the fact that my story isn't really unique. Every addict in there had parallel stories with an individual twist, no matter what their drug of choice happened to be.

I discussed my future with the head program counselor, who advised me not to test my sobriety and tempt fate by traveling to past party spots or frequenting old watering holes, as doing so often triggers a subconscious temptation to relapse. He also told me to get a sponsor and begin making regular appearances at AA. I nodded, smiled, and went off to pursue my sobriety on my terms.

I was determined to stay sober and make it last a lifetime. The early returns were positive and gave me incentive to keep going. I began losing weight and enjoyed waking up without feeling like death every morning. But lifetime habits are difficult to break, and learning to live a sober life, in my opinion, is the most difficult of all. It wasn't long before my lifetime habit took over once again.

With just three months of sobriety under my belt, I walked into a liquor store and bought a half gallon of Jägermeister and twelve-pack of beer on May 5, Cinco de Mayo. I wasn't celebrating the Mexican holiday, as I had many times in the past. I was simply sick of feeling like a fish out of water, trying to live a sober existence. Everything I did before always involved drinking, and now nothing did or could. Afternoons and evenings became huge, empty gaps of loneliness, anxiety, and depression. I enjoyed the socialization and good cheer of hanging out in bars and "getting my drink on," but all of that has to end when you get sober. In our treatment group, we were warned of "romanticizing" our drinking or dwelling on the "good old days" with our drinking buddies, except I wasn't going to a bar this time or going to drink with a friend. I was going home to drink alone, and I was about to ruin everything—again. I walked into that liquor store like I was on autopilot, but it felt like a death march at the same time. I dropped another fifty bucks on a product I knew was killing me and headed to the house for another evening of self-destruction.

I had always viewed treatment facilities as an absolute last resort and was quite certain that my drinking would never escalate to the point of having to go to one. The fact that it had now, indeed, gotten to that point, and that I had failed yet again to stay sober despite having gone to treatment, was very concerning. Although I had relapsed, my desire to stay away from the bottle remained. While admitting your problem is half the battle, the actual "not drinking" half proves to be more difficult.

CHAPTER 8

I LOVE YOU, MARY JANE

In the early 2010s, medical marijuana was making headlines and gaining legal traction throughout the country, including legalization in a few states. The reports were saying that cannabis was providing relief for a variety of conditions, including chronic pain, inflammation, anxiety, seizures, and PTSD. Almost daily news stories featured interviews with cancer patients, returning war veterans, and parents of epileptic children touting the benefits of cannabis and fighting for the right to use it.

I had smoked pot occasionally over the years, always when I was drunk or drinking. The psychoactive effect of marijuana on top of alcohol was often the "nail in the coffin" and led to bad experiences I preferred to avoid. I was taught growing up to stay away from drugs and not to associate with "potheads," as my mother called marijuana users. Alcohol was definitely my drug of choice, and it was socially acceptable everywhere.

Learning to live a sober life is like starting from scratch. Every method I had ever tried to quit drinking and get sober had failed. I was concerned about relapsing again and very intrigued by everything I was hearing and reading about cannabis. I eventually typed "medical marijuana for alcoholism" in a Google search, which was a life-changing event for me. The first article that I read was written by an alcoholic with a story hauntingly similar to mine who said that cannabis helped him quit drinking (see http://marijuana-uses.com/the-alcoholic-

51

fights-for-his-herb). The more I read, the more I wanted to know.

I learned about the history of cannabis in the United States, which was once a legal and thriving industry before becoming prohibited, as well as the very racist circumstances by which it became illegal. I watched video documentaries about alcoholics who claimed that cannabis helped them quit drinking and vastly improved their lives. This was a very exciting discovery, one that opened up an entirely new world for me. I decided that I was going to give it a try.

I wanted to buy some quality cannabis but needed a trusted source. I contacted a friend who, ironically, worked at the same liquor store where I spent thousands of dollars annually. I knew he smoked pot and asked him to get me some. I spent $100 for a quarter ounce of dank, dense nuggets and drove to a head shop, where I bought a small glass bong for $40. I didn't know how to roll a joint, but I had smoked bongs a few times in high school. The clerk at the head shop rang out the purchase and told me to "Have a good day!" I said "Thanks, this will help!"

Later that evening, while sitting in my recliner drinking a beer, I fired up a sample of the high-grade bud. The taste was incredible—a deep piney flavor—and came with an intense head rush followed by a complete body high. I felt like I was melting into my recliner. It was exceptionally enjoyable. I sent a text to the friend who sold it to me: "Wow!!!" I enjoyed getting stoned in the privacy of my home and experiencing the cannabis without being shitfaced. Although I was drinking on this particular evening, it became almost secondary to experimenting with the bud.

Over the next year, I continued to drink and smoke canna-bis, when I could get it. I quickly found another job and had income rolling in again. Cannabis seemed to help keep my drinking in check, as well as improve my appetite and quality of sleep. Complete abstinence was still my goal, but I definitely drank less—and felt healthier and happier—when I used can-nabis. I began to look forward to a hit from my bong after work as much as I always did a cold beer and shot.

I had several prescriptions that needed refilling and need-ed to address numerous health problems, so I scheduled an appointment with my doctor. I was open about my alcoholism and multiple attempts at sobriety, although I didn't mention that I had been using cannabis. She recommended a prescrip-tion drug called Campral that was supposed to reduce the craving for alcohol. After a clusterfuck of red tape convincing my insurance provider to pay for the alcohol cessation drug, I was finally able to get it filled. If anyone needed to try this, I did. In order for the drug to work properly, at least three weeks of abstinence was required prior to starting the medication.

I was ready to give sobriety another shot. The socializing and entertainment value of drinking—the reasons I started to drink in the first place—were long gone, replaced by multi-ple alcohol-related health problems and a very expensive habit to fund. Some months, the charges on my American Express card were more than $1,000 from my favorite bar alone, not to mention the cost of my liquor store arrangement and beer at the supermarket. My available cash was a fraction of what it once was, and I had long been outspending my income. Not only did my physical health depend on me putting the bottle down, but my financial health did as well. I sold the beloved Rolex I'd worn for more than ten years to Money Man Pawn for $3,500. I then went over to Purple Haze head shop, bought a big, beautiful glass bong, and still had a pocket full of cash left over.

I stopped drinking again and after three weeks of abstinence, I began taking the alcohol cessation medication, as instructed. My doctor told me that it could take a few weeks to start working, and I took it diligently. I continued using cannabis and was not only increasingly convinced of its medicinal benefits, but I was also quite certain it was helping me stay away from the bottle. To some, it may appear that is trading one addiction for another; however, this is a strategy called "Risk Reduction" therapy. The Risk Reduction method acknowledges that the use of one drug is acceptable when it reduces or eliminates the consumption of another, more harmful drug. It's a controversial approach and not advised by traditional substance abuse programs, but I've always gone against the grain and it was working well for me. I continued to research and absorb as much knowledge as possible about cannabis with the goal of becoming "self-sufficient."

I was eager to pick my brother's brain on growing cannabis. He has been smoking it since high school and learned how to grow it in the late '80s by reading *High Times* magazine. He told me that he hadn't bought weed since high school but smoked nearly every day. This was the type of self-sufficiency I was seeking, rather than the $400-per-ounce price tag I'd been paying. I wanted to learn how to produce my own unlimited supply and become an aficionado of all things cannabis.

I began purchasing the items I would need to grow my own cannabis. I continued watching videos, reading books, and learning as much about cannabis as time permitted. I became familiar with terms such as *terpenes* and *trichomes*, which describe the compounds that give each cannabis strain a unique fragrance, as well as the name of the resin heads that indicate when a bud is ripe. A few months later, I harvested my first cannabis plant. Although I made some mistakes along the way and ran into unexpected challenges, an answer was usually readily available with a quick internet search or in a gardening book. I was proud of my accomplishment and had several jars of decent cannabis for a fraction of the cost I had been paying. It is an extremely satisfying feeling to be able to grow your own medicine. It may not have been dispensary quality or looked like the cover bud on *High Times*, but it was more than adequate for my needs. I had found a new calling.

I continued taking the medication as directed and using cannabis. My cravings to drink seemed diminished, which is what the drug is intended to do, but I also felt that the cannabis reduced my urge to drink. After more than thirty years of hard partying that nearly killed me and thousands of failed attempts to quit drinking, it seemed that I was finally on the right path.

CHAPTER 9

TURNING OVER A NEW LEAF

I had been sober for a few months and had lost ten or fifteen pounds without doing anything other than staying away from booze and smoking weed. I was sleeping soundly and waking up feeling good. The weight loss was noticeable to others and made my pants so loose I had to go down a size. It was a great feeling.

Unfortunately, ongoing pain in my knee was getting unbearable, and after several years of steroid injections, I needed a total knee replacement at age forty-five. Days before the surgery, I purchased a cane at a drugstore and was also using my father's walker to get around. Putting it off any further wasn't an option.

The procedure went well, and my surgeon told me that my knee had been bone-on-bone arthritic. As the fog lifted and pain came on in strong, intensifying waves, I was real glad to have chosen the narcotic option. The first time trying to walk down the hall was excruciating. I felt helpless needing assistance walking to the bathroom and ridiculous wearing a hospital gown. After a few days, I was doing somewhat better and was discharged. I was looking forward to going home and recovering in my recliner with my pain meds and plenty of homegrown.

As my knee was recovering from the surgery, my reliance on a cane remained. The lack of sensation and weakness in my legs and feet were much greater than before, and I'd easily lose my balance. I felt like I was walking with heavy ankle weights on and had been tripping a lot, which I initially attributed to certain shoes or clumsiness. I later learned that this is a symptom of alcoholic neuropathy called "foot drop." I had some incidents when driving where I would lose orientation of my foot placement and couldn't tell if it was on the accelerator or the brake—or I'd be on both at the same time and nearly run into the car in front of me. After a series of episodes like this, I made an appointment with a neurologist to confirm what I already suspected.

The neurologist performed a nerve conduction study and an EMG test that indicated severe, permanent alcoholic neuropathy. He said it was the worst case he had ever seen in a patient who wasn't diabetic and asked why I drank so much. I told him I was an alcoholic but didn't drink anymore. It felt strange saying those words to a stranger, but they felt good to say. He told me that the damage was irreversible and that I should start riding a stationary bike to slow further muscle loss. I asked about driving, and in a loud, firm voice, he said, "I don't know how you can drive a car!" He sounded irritated that I'd asked such a stupid question. A short time later, I stopped driving after continued incidents of foot disorientation and near misses while behind the wheel.

Around the same time, I'd been communicating with a guy from high school who confided in me about his struggle with alcoholism. I private-messaged him a few times, telling him how I'd been using cannabis instead of drinking and that it had been working well for me. He said he respected that but that cannabis wasn't his thing, and then he signed off to meet a friend for an AA meeting. I sent a reply and noticed the next day that he hadn't read it until 2:30 a.m. I silently suspected that he may have gone off the wagon after his AA meeting, if he even made it there at all. A day or two later, I received news that he was found dead after drinking all night. He drank himself to death.

While this news and the findings of my neurologist were a shocking, double punch to the gut, I also felt blessed that I was still alive, considering the abuse I'd put my body throughout my life. For a long time, I was quite certain that I would likely die of cirrhosis or liver cancer and purposely avoided getting blood work that would indicate such. I often had discomfort in my upper-right abdomen, which I later learned was a swollen, fatty liver. I even used to say on occasion, "At least I know what I'm gonna die from." Fortunately, my once off-the-charts liver and pancreatic enzymes had returned to normal, and even though I had permanent nerve damage, I felt like I had a new start on life at the same time.

I began making a purposeful, conscious effort to live a healthier, happier life and to treat each day as a gift. I wanted to become leaner and stronger, and I figured that this was probably the best opportunity and most incentive I'd ever had to do so. Rather than announce my weight loss and fitness goals on Facebook to "friends" I barely knew, I decided that social media was a distraction I no longer wanted and deleted my accounts. By doing so, I gained plenty of time for exercise. I began incorporating healthier eating habits, starting with a daily breakfast of Greek yogurt and a banana with peanut butter, instead of eating previous night's heavy leftovers, which I'd been doing for years. I also started eliminating processed foods from my diet and eating an apple after dinner each night. These small, simple changes upped my fiber and fruit intake while drastically reducing the overall number of calories I'd been consuming.

I had lost a significant amount of weight after my first divorce, and I wanted to do it again. I started taking short walks and riding a stationary bike, as my neurologist suggested. I bought a forty-pound dumbbell set and incline bench to start lifting weights. I hadn't lifted weights at all since my DUI arrest twenty years earlier, usually because working out with a hangover was always misery. Since I was no longer drinking, I no longer had that obstacle. I put together a beginner's weight routine and started with one set of each exercise. I eventually progressed to three and four sets and began adding pull-ups as well. If I couldn't complete a full workout as I planned, I did what I was able to do, and the persistence paid off. About nine months after I quit drinking, I had lost about sixty pounds and had better muscle tone than I'd had in years.

CHAPTER 10

FLEEING PARADISE

With more than fifty people per day continuing to move to Charleston, and with no end in sight, traffic and density first became a nuisance then a regular problem. Gridlock is a daily occurrence, as well as "sunny day" flooding and extreme weather events. The high cost of homeowner and flood insurance premiums continue to rise as storms become stronger and coastal construction costs soar. One only need look at their insurance premium to determine their risk of catastrophe; insurance companies are experts at doing that.

Charleston loves its booze, and drunkenness is not just accepted but often expected. Any large events or festivals held in the Holy City often become drunken free-for-alls and traffic nightmares—the annual Boone Hall Oyster Festival is a perfect example. Cannabis, on the other hand, remains taboo and highly illegal. South Carolina is far behind most other states when it comes to cannabis legalization, and penalties are severe for mere possession of a joint. As a recovering alcoholic who uses cannabis daily for alcohol abstinence, anxiety, depression, and glaucoma, I no longer wanted to risk draconian incarceration for relief. My gut told me that legal ganja at the City Market or on King Street anytime soon seemed far-fetched, so it was time to go.

We decided to move north, to an area that I once couldn't wait to get away from. It's a quiet, rural farming community where people's yards are measured in acres and surrounded by cornfields. There is little traffic, unlike Charleston, and it's a refreshing change to being able to reach out and touch your neighbor. When we announced our move to family and friends, we heard our fair share of snow and cold weather jokes. I kindly reminded them, though, that when the winters are cold and snowy, we will simply stay indoors by a warm, cozy fire and have no need to flee. The same cannot be said about the potential for total devastation from hurricanes that threaten the coast each summer and continue to get stronger.

I've been sober since 2014, but I still think about drinking every day. It was only a few years ago since I was planted at a barstool every afternoon, but it feels like an eternity. Not long ago, a life without alcohol seemed inconceivable. It was devoured in celebration and sadness, in good times and bad, or for no reason at all. It was there at the end of every workday and at the start of many mornings. It had been my constant companion since I was a teenager, and the notion of missing even a single day of drinking caused great anxiety.

When I was younger, I always had to be where all the action was so I could "see and be seen." None of that matters to me anymore, and I now live a very quiet and private life. I think about when I'd stumble home drunk in the middle of the night and nearly burn the house down after passing out with a pizza in the oven, or waking up on the couch with food spilled all over my clothes and a broken plate on the floor. It was all part of the life then, but it embarrasses me greatly now.

I've often wondered if those officers had arrested me that early morning when I was seventeen, seeing double and unable to stand on my own, if my life would have turned out differently. I realize now that drinking always amplified life's crises and blurred my best options. My mom used to tell me, "When you keep doing what you've been doing, you're going to keep getting what you've been getting." I kept walking into a wall for thirty years, and then I'd back up and do it over and over again, never accepting that drinking was the root of my problems.

My dad quit drinking in his mid-forties and often encouraged me to quit too. "You know how good you feel when you haven't had a drink for a few days?" he used to say. "That's just the tip of the iceberg. It only gets better and better." He was elated that I had quit drinking. He'd told me that he and my mother were worried they'd have to bury me one day if I continued going like I was. Although I was never convinced at the time, I can absolutely attest that my life has improved immensely since I removed alcohol, and I'm glad he was able to finally see me do it.

I've always been the captain of my own ship, even when it's sinking, and I've lived a unique life. I've had more than three dozen jobs in my life, quit them all except two, and yet made more money by age thirty-five than many people do in a lifetime. I've butchered meat, sold groceries, driven forklifts, catered weddings, managed hotels, supervised staff, built cars, parked cars, carried luggage, and stocked shelves. I've patrolled streets, performed traffic stops, made arrests, and taken people to jail. I've traveled to more than a dozen different countries and have flown on hundreds of flights, including first class and chartered aircraft. I have a two-year degree that took me six years to earn in a field I never should have pursued. I've been married three times and divorced twice, but my third wife has been my charm.

I've come to realize that my continual quest to chase the "greener grass on the other side of the fence" was never really about money or job title. It was about finding the "perfect" job that would coexist with my alcohol habit. In my eyes, an employer should have allowed me to call off when I was hungover, be lenient if I was late, and tolerant of shitty performance. It meant that they should ignore the previous night's booze on my breath and be understanding of requests for time off or frequent "emergencies" that required my absence. To me, a job was simply a way to make money to pay my bills and buy booze. I took for granted the ability to earn an income and burned most bridges I've ever set foot on.

Becoming sober is my biggest life accomplishment. I don't go to meetings and have never had a sponsor. I became a self-sustaining cannabis farmer, advocate, and enthusiast, and I firmly believe that it saved my life. It is the best "job" I've ever had; the compensation is relief, sobriety, and life, not money. I am a Cannabist.

ABOUT THE AUTHOR

My journey to an alcohol-free existence has been long and difficult, as well as on a path less traveled, but it has very much been worth the effort. I hope that my story and this book will contribute to the global legalization of cannabis, as well as inspire others to take responsibility for their health and well-being. There really is truth in the saying, "You reap what you sow."

poisoned_pirate@pm.me

Made in the USA
Monee, IL
15 June 2021

71418053R00046